The Easy and Complete Dash Diet Plan

Tasty and Fast Recipes
for a Better Diet Plan

Eleonore Barlow

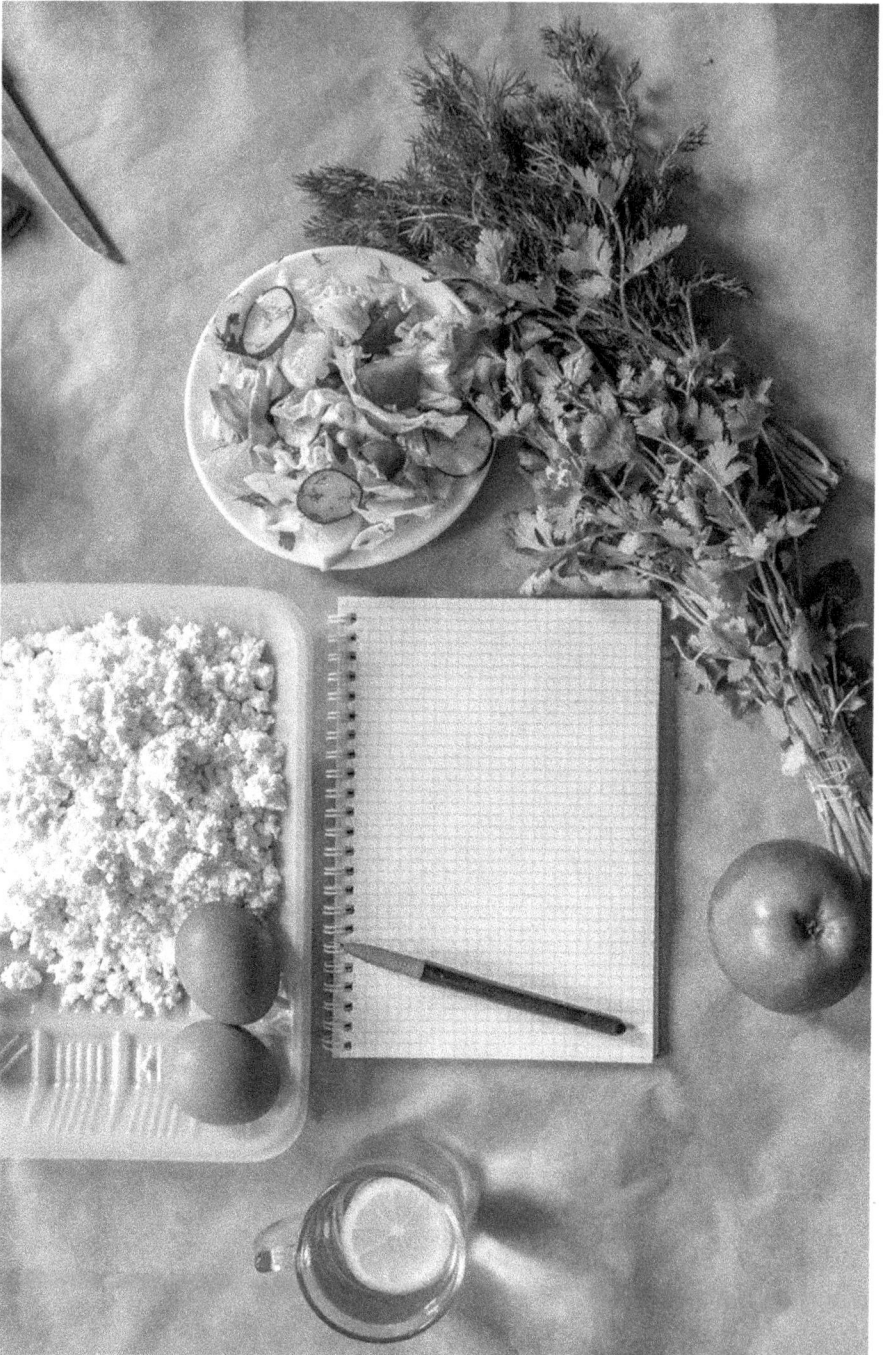

Table of Contents

Basil and Tomato Baked Eggs

Serving: 2

Prep Time: 10 minutes

Cook Time: 15 minutes

Ingredients:

1/2 garlic clove, minced

1/2 cup canned tomatoes

¼ cup fresh basil leaves, roughly chopped 1/4 teaspoon chili powder 1/2 tablespoon olive oil

2 whole eggs

Pepper to taste

How To:

1.   Preheat your oven to 375 degrees F.

2.   Take alittle baking dish and grease with vegetable oil .

3.   Add garlic, basil, tomatoes chili, vegetable oil into a dish and stir.

4.   Crack eggs into a dish, keeping space between the 2 .

6

5.   Sprinkle the entire dish with sunflower seeds and pepper.

6.   Place in oven and cook for 12 minutes until eggs are set and tomatoes are bubbling.

7.   Serve with basil on top.

Enjoy!

Nutrition (Per Serving)

Calories: 235

Fat: 16g

Carbohydrates: 7g

Protein: 14g

Cool Mushroom Munchies

Serving: 2

Prep Time: 5 minutes

Cook Time: 10 minutes

Ingredients:

4 Portobello mushroom caps

3 tablespoons coconut aminos

2 tablespoons sesame oil

1 tablespoon fresh ginger, minced

1 small garlic clove, minced

How To:

1.   Set your broiler to low, keeping the rack 6 inches from the heating source.

2.   Wash mushrooms under cold water and transfer them to a baking sheet (top side down).

3.   Take a bowl and blend in vegetable oil , garlic, coconut aminos, ginger and pour the mixture over the mushrooms tops .

4.   Cook for 10 minutes.

5.   Serve and enjoy!

Nutrition (Per Serving)

Calories: 196

Fat: 14g

Carbohydrates: 14g

Protein: 7g

Banana and Buckwheat Porridge

Serving: 2

Prep Time: 10 minutes

Cook Time: 15 minutes

Ingredients:

1 cup of water

1 cup buckwheat groats

2 big grapefruits, peeled and sliced

1 tablespoon ground cinnamon

3-4 cups almond milk

2 tablespoons natural almond butter

How To:

1. Take a medium-sized saucepan and add buckwheat and water.

2. Place the pan over medium heat and convey to a boil.

3. Keep cooking until the buckwheat absorbs the water.

4.   Reduce heat to low and add almond milk, stir gently.

5.   Add the remainder of the ingredients (except the grapefruits).

6.   Stir and take away from the warmth.

7.   Transfer into cereal bowls and add grapefruit chunks.

8.   Serve and enjoy!

Nutrition (Per Serving)

Calories: 223

Fat: 4g

Carbohydrates: 4g

Protein: 7g

Delightful Berry Quinoa Bowl

Serving: 4

Prep Time: 5 minutes

Cook Time: 15 minutes

Ingredients:

1 cup quinoa

2 cups of water

1 piece, 2-inch sized cinnamon stick

2-3 tablespoons of maple syrup

Flavorful Toppings

½ cup blueberries, raspberries or strawberries

2 tablespoons raisins

1 teaspoon lime

¼ teaspoon nutmeg, grated

3 tablespoons whipped coconut cream

2 tablespoon cashew nuts, chopped

How To:

1.   Take a metal strainer and pass your grain through them to strain them well.

2.   Rinse the grains under cold water thoroughly.

3.   Take a medium-sized saucepan and pour within the water.

4.   Add the strained grains and convey the entire mixture to a boil.

5.   Add cinnamon sticks and canopy the saucepan.

6.   Lower the warmth and let the mixture simmer for quarter-hour to permit the grain to soak up the liquid.

7.   Remove the warmth and plump up the mixture employing a fork.

8.   Add syrup if you would like additional flavor.

9.   Also, if you're looking to form things a touch more interesting, just add any of the abovementioned ingredients.

Nutrition (Per Serving)

Calories: 202

Fat: 5g

Carbohydrates: 35g

Protein: 6g

Protein: 1.4g

Fantastic Bowl of Steel Oats

Serving: 4

Prep Time: 5 minutes

Cook Time: 25 minutes

Ingredients:

3 ¾ cup water

1 ¼ cup steel-cut oats

¼ teaspoon salt

Flavorful Toppings

1 teaspoon cinnamon

½ teaspoon nutmeg

½ teaspoon lemon pepper

1 teaspoon Garam masala

Mixed berries as needed

Diced mangos as needed

Sliced bananas as needed

Dried fruits as needed

Nuts as needed

Flavorful Toppings

1 tablespoon coconut milk

How To:

1.   Take a medium-sized saucepan and convey it over high heat.

2.   Add water and permit the water to heat up.

3.   Add the steel-cut oats with some salt and lower the warmth to medium-low.

4.   Let the mixture simmer for about 25 minutes, ensuring to stay stirring it all the way.

5.   Add coconut milk or almond butter for a few extra flavor.

6.   Once done, serve with some berries or nuts.

7.   Enjoy!

Nutrition (Per Serving)

Calories: 125

Fat: 3g

Carbohydrates: 20g

Protein: 7g

Quinoa and Cinnamon Bowl

Serving: 2

Prep Time: 10 minutes

Cook Time: 15 minutes

Ingredients:

1 cup uncooked quinoa

1½ cups water

½ teaspoon ground cinnamon

½ teaspoon sunflower seeds

A drizzle of almond/coconut milk for serving

How To:

1.   Rinse quinoa thoroughly underwater.

2.   Take a medium-sized saucepan and add quinoa, water, cinnamon, and seeds.

3.   Stir and place it over medium-high heat.

4.   Bring the combination to a boil.

5.   Reduce heat to low and simmer for 10 minutes.

6.   Once cooked, remove from the warmth and let it cool.

7.   Serve with a drizzle of almond or coconut milk.

8.   Enjoy!

Nutrition (Per Serving)

Calories: 255

Fat: 13g

Carbohydrates: 33g

Protein: 5g

Awesome Breakfast Parfait

Serving: 2

Prep Time: 5 minutes

Cook Time: Nil

Ingredients:

1 teaspoon sunflower seeds

½ cup low-fat milk

1 cup all-purpose flour

1 teaspoon vanilla

3 eggs, beaten

1 teaspoon baking soda

2 cups non-fat Greek yogurt

How To:

1.   Hack pretzels into small-sized portions and slice the strawberries.

2.   Add yogurt to rock bottom of the glass and top with pretzel pieces and strawberries.

3.   Add more yogurt and keep repeating until you've got spent all the ingredients.

4.   Enjoy!

Nutrition (Per Serving)

Calorie: 304

Fat: 1g

Carbohydrates: 58g

Protein: 15g

Golden Eggplant Fries

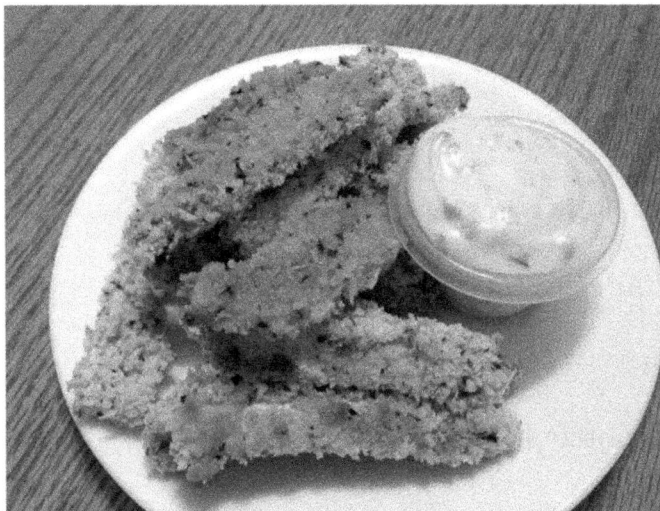

Serving: 8

Prep Time: 10 minutes

Cook Time: 15 minutes

Ingredients:

2 eggs

2 cups almond flour

2 tablespoons coconut oil, spray

2 eggplant, peeled and cut thinly Sunflower seeds and pepper

How To:

1.   Preheat your oven to 400 degrees F.

2.   Take a bowl and blend with sunflower seeds and black pepper.

3.   Take another bowl and beat eggs until frothy.

4.   Dip the eggplant pieces into the eggs.

5.   Then coat them with the flour mixture.

6.   Add another layer of flour and egg.

7.   Then, take a baking sheet and grease with copra oil on top.

8.   Bake for about quarter-hour.

9.   Serve and enjoy!

Nutrition (Per Serving)

Calories: 212

Fat: 15.8g

Carbohydrates: 12.1g

Protein: 8.6g

Traditional Black Bean Chili

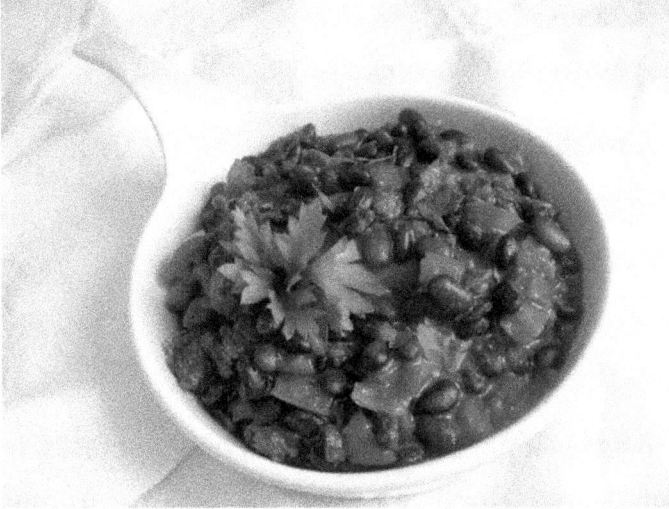

Serving: 4

Prep Time: 10 minutes

Cooking Time: 4 hours

Ingredients:

1 ½ cups red bell pepper, chopped

1 cup yellow onion, chopped

1 ½ cups mushrooms, sliced

1 tablespoon olive oil

1 tablespoon chili powder

2 garlic cloves, minced

1 teaspoon chipotle chili pepper, chopped ½ teaspoon cumin, ground

16 ounces canned black beans, drained and rinsed

2 tablespoons cilantro, chopped

1 cup tomatoes, chopped

How To:

1.   Add red bell peppers, onion, dill, mushrooms, flavor, garlic, chili pepper, cumin, black beans, tomatoes to your Slow Cooker.

2.   Stir well.

3.   Place lid and cook on HIGH for 4 hours.

4.   Sprinkle cilantro on top.

5.   Serve and enjoy!

Nutrition (Per Serving)

Calories: 211

Fat: 3g

Carbohydrates: 22g

Protein: 5g

Very Wild Mushroom Pilaf

Serving: 4

Prep Time: 10 minutes

Cooking Time: 3 hours

Ingredients:

1 cup wild rice

2 garlic cloves, minced

6 green onions, chopped

2 tablespoons olive oil

½ pound baby Bella mushrooms

2 cups water

How To:

1.   Add rice, garlic, onion, oil, mushrooms and water to your Slow Cooker.

2.   Stir well until mixed.

3.   Place lid and cook on LOW for 3 hours.

4.   Stir pilaf and divide between serving platters.

5.   Enjoy!

Nutrition (Per Serving)

Calories: 210

Fat: 7g

Carbohydrates: 16g

Protein: 4g

Green Palak Paneer

Serving: 4

Prep Time: 5 minutes

Cook Time: 10 minutes

Ingredients:

1-pound spinach

2 cups cubed paneer (vegan)

2 tablespoons coconut oil

1 tcaspoon cumin

1 chopped up onion

1-2 teaspoons hot green chili minced up

1 teaspoon minced garlic

15 cashews

4 tablespoons almond milk

1 teaspoon Garam masala

Flavored vinegar as needed

How To:

1.   Add cashews and milk to a blender and blend well.

2.   Set your pot to Sauté mode and add coconut oil; allow the oil to heat up.

3.   Add cumin seeds, garlic, green chilies, ginger and sauté for 1 minute.

4.   Add onion and sauté for two minutes.

5.   Add chopped spinach, flavored vinegar and a cup of water.

6.   Lock up the lid and cook on high for 10 minutes.

7.   Quick-release the pressure.

8.   Add ½ cup of water and blend to a paste.

9.   Add cashew paste, paneer and Garam Masala and stir thoroughly.

10.   Serve over hot rice!

Nutrition (Per Serving)

Calories: 367
Fat: 26g
Carbohydrates: 21g
Protein: 16g

Sporty Baby Carrots

Serving: 4

Prep Time: 5 minutes

Cook Time: 5 minutes

Ingredients:

1-pound baby carrots

1 cup water

1 tablespoon clarified ghee

1 tablespoon chopped up fresh mint leaves Sea flavored vinegar as needed

How To:

1. Place a steamer rack on top of your pot and add the carrots.

2. Add water.

3. Lock the lid and cook at high for two minutes.

4. Do a fast release.

5. Pass the carrots through a strainer and drain them.

6. Wipe the insert clean.

7. Return the insert to the pot and set the pot to Sauté mode.

8. Add drawn butter and permit it to melt.

9. Add mint and sauté for 30 seconds.

10. Add carrots to the insert and sauté well.

11. Remove them and sprinkle with little bit of flavored vinegar on top.

12. Enjoy!

Nutrition (Per Serving)

Calories: 131

Fat: 10g

Carbohydrates: 11g

Protein: 1g

Almond Butter Pork Chops

Serving: 2

Prep Time: 5 minutes

Cook Time: 25 minutes

Ingredients:

1 tablespoon almond butter, divided

2 boneless pork chops

Pepper to taste

1 tablespoon dried Italian seasoning, low fat and low sodium

1 tablespoon olive oil

How To:

1.   Pre-heat your oven to 350 degrees F.

2.   Pat pork chops dry with a towel and place them during a baking dish.

3.   Season with pepper, and Italian seasoning.

4.   Drizzle vegetable oil over pork chops.

5. Top each chop with ½ tablespoon almond butter.

6. Bake for 25 minutes.

7. Transfer pork chops on two plates and top with almond butter juice.

8. Serve and enjoy!

Nutrition (Per Serving)

Calories: 333

Fat: 23g

Carbohydrates: 1g

Protein: 31g

Chicken Salsa

Serving: 1

Prep Time: 4 minutes

Cook Time: 14 minutes

Ingredients:

2 chicken breasts

1 cup salsa

1 taco seasoning mix

1 cup plain Greek Yogurt

½ cup of kite ricottta/cashew cheese, cubed

How To:

1.   Take a skillet and place over medium heat.

2.   Add pigeon breast, ½ cup of salsa and taco seasoning.

3.   Mix well and cook for 12-15 minutes until the chicken is completed.

4.   Take the back off and cube them.

5.   Place the cubes on toothpick and top with cheddar.

6.   Place yogurt and remaining salsa in cups and use as dips.

7. Enjoy!

Nutrition (Per Serving)

Calories: 359

Fat: 14g

Net Carbohydrates: 14g

Protein: 43g

Healthy Mediterranean Lamb Chops

Serving: 4

Prep Time: 10 minutes

Cook Time: 10 minutes

Ingredients:

4 lamb shoulder chops, 8 ounces each

2 tablespoons Dijon mustard

2 tablespoons Balsamic vinegar

½ cup olive oil

2 tablespoons shredded fresh basil

How To:

1.   Pat your lamb chop dry employing a kitchen towel and arrange them on a shallow glass baking dish.

2.   Take a bowl and a whisk in Dijon mustard, balsamic vinegar, pepper and blend them well.

3.   Whisk within the oil very slowly into the marinade until the mixture is smooth

4. Stir in basil.

5. Pour the marinade over the lamb chops and stir to coat each side well.

6. Cover the chops and permit them to marinate for 1-4 hours (chilled).

7. Take the chops out and leave them for half-hour to permit the temperature to succeed in a traditional level.

8. Pre-heat your grill to medium heat and add oil to the grate.

9. Grill the lamb chops for 5-10 minutes per side until each side are browned.

10. Once the middle reads 145 degrees F, the chops are ready, serve and enjoy!

Nutrition (Per Serving)

Calories: 521

Fat: 45g

Carbohydrates: 3.5g

Protein: 22g

Amazing Sesame Breadsticks

Serving: 5 breadsticks

Prep Time: 10 minutes

Cooking Time: 20 minutes

Ingredients:

1 egg white

2 tablespoons almond flour

1 teaspoon Himalayan pink sunflower seeds

1 tablespoon extra-virgin olive oil

½ teaspoon sesame seeds

How To:

1.   Pre-heat your oven to 320 degrees F.

2.   Line a baking sheet with parchment paper and keep it on the side.

3.   Take a bowl and whisk in egg whites, add flour and half sunflower seeds and vegetable oil.

4.   Knead until you've got a smooth dough.

5.   Divide into 4 pieces and roll into breadsticks.

6.   Place on prepared sheet and brush with vegetable oil , sprinkle sesame seeds and remaining sunflower seeds.

7.   Bake for 20 minutes.

8.   Serve and enjoy!

Nutrition (Per Serving)

Total Carbs: 1.1g

Fiber: 1g

Protein: 1.6g

Fat: 5g

Cucumber and Zucchini Soup

Serving: 3

Prep Time: 10 minutes + Chill time

Cook Time: nil

Ingredients:

2 tablespoons olive oil

1 tablespoon fresh dill

2/5 cup fresh cream

7 ounces cucumber, cubed

10 ½ zucchini, cubed

1 red pepper, chopped

3 celery stalks, chopped

Sunflower seeds and pepper to taste

How To:

1.   Add all the veggies during a juice and make a smooth juice.

2.   Mix within the fresh cream and vegetable oil.

3.   Season with pepper and sunflower seeds.

4.   Garnish with dill.

5.   Serve chilled and enjoy!

Nutrition (Per Serving)

Calories: 100

Fat: 8g

Carbohydrates: 4g

Protein: 2g

Crockpot Pumpkin Soup

Serving: 3

Prep Time: 10 minutes

Cook Time: 6-8 hours

Ingredients:

1 small pumpkin, halved, peeled, seeds removed, and pulp cubed

2 cups chicken broth

1 cup of coconut almond milk

Sunflower seeds, pepper, thyme, and pepper, to taste

How To:

1.   Add all the ingredients to a crockpot.

2.   Close the lid.

3.   Cook for 6-8 hours on LOW.

4.   Make a smooth puree by employing a blender.

5.   Garnish with roasted seeds.

6.   Serve and enjoy!

Nutrition (Per Serving)

Calories: 60

Fat: 5g

Carbohydrates: 4g

Protein: 4g

Tomato Soup

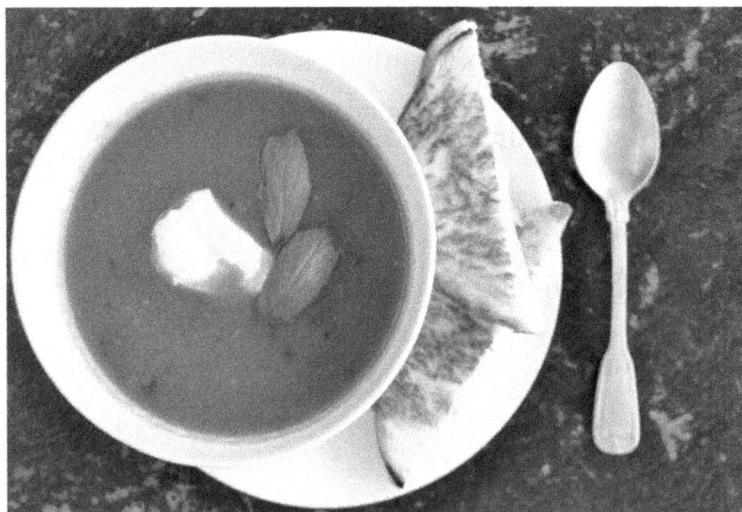

Serving: 3

Prep Time: 10 minutes

Cook Time: 6-8 hours

Ingredients:

4 cups water or vegetable broth

7 large tomatoes, ripe

½ cup macadamia nuts, raw

1 medium onion, chopped

Sunflower seeds and pepper to taste

How To:

1.   Take a nonstick skillet and add the onion.

2.   Brown the onion for five minutes.

3.   Add all the ingredients to a crockpot.

4.   Cook for 6-8 hours on LOW.

5.   Make a smooth puree by employing a blender.

6.   Serve it warm and enjoy!

Nutrition (Per Serving)

Calories: 145

Fat: 12g

Carbohydrates: 8g

Protein: 6g

Pumpkin, Coconut and Sage Soup

Serving: 3

Prep Time: 10 minutes

Cook Time: 30 minutes

Ingredients:

1 cup pumpkin, canned

6 cups chicken broth

1 cup low fat coconut almond milk

1 teaspoon sage, chopped

3 garlic cloves, peeled

Sunflower seeds and pepper to taste

How To:

1.   Take a stockpot and add all the ingredients except coconut almond milk into it.

2.   Place stockpot over medium heat.

3.   Let it bring back a boil.

4. Reduce heat to simmer for half-hour.

5. Add the coconut almond milk and stir.

6. Serve bacon and enjoy!

Nutrition (Per Serving)

Calories: 145

Fat: 12g

Carbohydrates: 8g

Protein: 6g

Sweet Potato and Leek Soup

Serving: 6

Prep Time: 10 minutes

Cook Time: 8 hours

Ingredients:

6 cups sweet potatoes, peeled and cubed

2 leeks, whites and greens, sliced

6 cups vegetable stock

1 teaspoon dried thyme

1 teaspoon salt

¼ teaspoon fresh ground black pepper

How To:

1.   Add sweet potatoes, leeks, thyme, stock, salt and pepper to your Slow Cooker.

2.   Close lid and cook on LOW for 8 hours.

3.   Mash with potato masher/ use an immersion blender to smooth the soup.

4.   Serve and enjoy!

Nutrition (Per Serving)

Calories: 234

Fat: 2g

Carbohydrates: 47g

Protein: 8g

The Kale and Spinach Soup

Serving: 4

Prep Time: 5 minutes

Cook Time: 10 minutes

Ingredients:

3 ounces coconut oil

8 ounces kale, chopped

2 avocados, diced

4 1/3 cups coconut almond milk

Sunflower seeds and pepper to taste

How To:

1.   Take a skillet and place it over medium heat. 2. Add kale and sauté for 2-3 minutes

2.   Add kale to blender.

3.   Add water, spices, coconut almond milk and avocado to blender also.

4.   Blend until smooth and pour mix into bowl.

5.   Serve and enjoy!

Nutrition (Per Serving)

Calories: 124

Fat: 13g

Carbohydrates: 7g

Protein: 4.2g

Japanese Onion Soup

Serving: 4

Prep Time: 15 minutes

Cook Time: 45 minutes

Ingredients:

½ stalk celery, diced

1 small onion, diced

½ carrot, diced

1 teaspoon fresh ginger root, grated

¼ teaspoon fresh garlic, minced

2 tablespoons chicken stock

3 teaspoons beef bouillon granules

1 cup fresh shiitake, mushrooms

2 quarts water

1 cup baby Portobello mushrooms, sliced

1 tablespoon fresh chives

How To:

1.   Take a saucepan and place it over high heat, add water, bring back a boil.

2.   Add beef bouillon, celery, onion, chicken broth, carrots, half the mushrooms, ginger, garlic.

3.   placed on the lid and reduce heat to medium, cook for 45 minutes.

4.   Take another saucepan and add another half mushroom.

5.   Once the soup is cooked, strain the soup into the pot with uncooked mushrooms.

6.   Garnish with chives and enjoy!

Nutrition (Per Serving)

Calories: 25

Fat: 0.2g

Carbohydrates: 5g

Protein: 1.4g

Amazing Broccoli and Cauliflower Soup

Serving: 4

Prep Time: 10 minutes

Cooking Time: 8 hours

Ingredients:

3 cups broccoli florets

2 cups cauliflower florets

2 garlic cloves, minced

½ cup shallots, chopped

1 carrot, chopped

3 ½ cups low sodium veggie stick

Pinch of pepper

1 cup fat-free milk

6 ounces low-fat cheddar, shredded

1 cup non-fat Greek yogurt

How To:

1.   Add broccoli, cauliflower, garlic, shallots, carrot, stock, pepper to your Slow Cooker.

2.   Stir well and place lid.

3.   Cook on LOW for 8 hours.

4.   Add milk and cheese.

5.   Use an immersion blender to smooth the soup.

6.   Add yogurt and blend another time.

7.   Ladle into bowls and enjoy!

Nutrition (Per Serving)

Calories: 218

Fat: 11g

Carbohydrates: 15g

Protein: 12g

Amazing Zucchini Soup

Serving: 4

Prep Time: 10 minutes

Cook Time: 20 minutes

Ingredients:

1 onion, chopped

3 zucchini, cut into medium chunks

2 tablespoons coconut milk

2 garlic cloves, minced

4 cups chicken stock

2 tablespoons coconut oil

Pinch of salt

Black pepper to taste

How To:

1.   Take a pot and place over medium heat.

2.   Add oil and let it heat up.

3.   Add zucchini, garlic, onion and stir.

4.   Cook for five minutes.

5.   Add stock, salt, pepper and stir.

6.   bring back a boil and reduce the warmth.

7.   Simmer for 20 minutes.

8.   Remove from heat and add coconut milk.

9.   Use an immersion blender until smooth.

10.   Ladle into soup bowls and serve.

11.   Enjoy!

Nutrition (Per Serving)

Calories: 160

Fat: 2g

Carbohydrates: 4g

Protein: 7g

Spanish Mussels

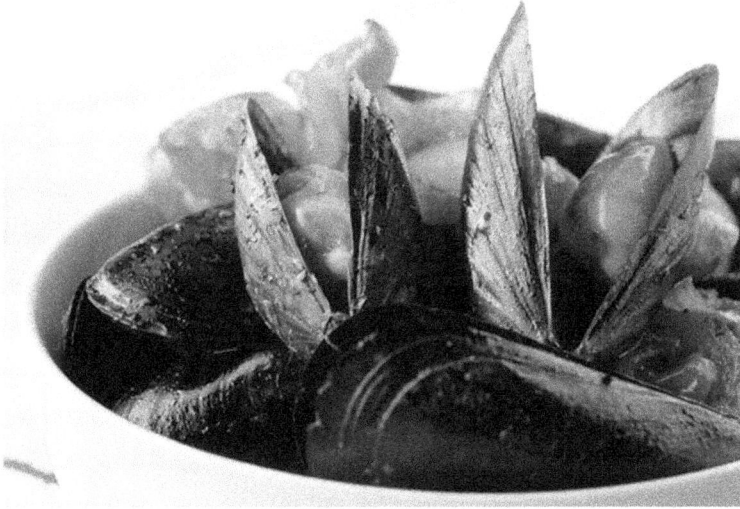

Serving: 4

Prep Time: 10 minutes

Cook Time: 23 minutes

Ingredients:

tablespoons olive oil

pounds mussels, scrubbed

Pepper to taste

cups canned tomatoes, crushed

shallot, chopped

garlic cloves, minced

cups low sodium vegetable stock

1/3 cup cilantro, chopped

How To:

1.   Take a pan and place it over medium-high heat, add shallot and stir-cook for 3 minutes.

2.   Add garlic, stock, tomatoes, pepper, stir and reduce heat, simmer for 10 minutes.

3.   Add mussels, cilantro, and toss.

4.   Cover and cook for 10 minutes more.

5.   Serve and enjoy!

Nutrition (Per Serving)

Calories: 210

Fat: 2g

Carbohydrates: 5g

Protein: 8g

Tilapia Broccoli Platter

Serving: 2

Prep Time: 4 minutes

Cook Time: 14 minutes

Ingredients:

Ounce tilapia, frozen

1 tablespoon almond butter

1 tablespoon garlic, minced

1 teaspoon lemon pepper seasoning

1 cup broccoli florets, fresh

How To:

1.   Pre-heat your oven to 350 degrees F.

2.   Add fish in aluminum foil packets.

3.   Arrange broccoli around fish.

4.   Sprinkle lemon pepper on top.

5.   Close the packets and seal.

6.   Bake for 14 minutes.

7.   Take a bowl and add garlic and almond butter, mix well and keep the mixture on the side.

8.   Remove the packet from oven and transfer to platter.

9.   Place almond butter on top of the fish and broccoli, serve and enjoy!

Nutrition (Per Serving)

Calories: 362

Fat: 25g

Carbohydrates: 2g

Protein: 29g

Salmon with Peas and Parsley Dressing

Serving: 4

Prep Time: 15 minutes

Cook Time: 15 minutes

Ingredients:

16 ounces salmon fillets, boneless and skin-on

1 tablespoon parsley, chopped

10 ounces peas

9 ounces vegetable stock, low sodium

2 cups water

½ teaspoon oregano, dried

½ teaspoon sweet paprika

2 garlic cloves, minced

A pinch of black pepper

How To:

1.   Add garlic, parsley, paprika, oregano and stock to a kitchen appliance and blend.

2.   Add water to your Instant Pot.

3.   Add steam basket.

4.   Add fish fillets inside the steamer basket.

5.   Season with pepper.

6.   Lock the lid and cook on high for 10 minutes.

7.   Release the pressure naturally over 10 minutes .

8.   Divide the fish amongst plates.

9.   Add peas to the steamer basket and lock the lid again, cook on high for five minutes.

10.   Quick release the pressure.

11.   Divide the peas next to your fillets and serve with the parsley dressing drizzled

12.   on top

13.   Enjoy!

Nutrition (Per Serving)

Calories: 315

Fat: 5g

Carbohydrates: 14g

Protein: 16g

Mackerel and Orange Medley

Serving: 4

Prep Time: 10 minutes

Cook Time: 10 minutes

Ingredients:

mackerel fillets, skinless and boneless

spring onion, chopped

1 teaspoon olive oil

1-inch ginger piece, grated

Black pepper as needed

Juice and zest of 1 whole orange

1 cup low sodium fish stock

How To:

1.   Season the fillets with black pepper and rub vegetable oil .

2.   Add stock, fruit juice , ginger, orange peel and onion to Instant Pot.

3.   Place a steamer basket and add the fillets.

4.   Lock the lid and cook on high for 10 minutes.

5.   Release the pressure naturally over 10 minutes.

6.   Divide the fillets amongst plates and drizzle the orange sauce from the pot over the fish.

7.   Enjoy!

Nutrition (Per Serving)

Calories: 200

Fat: 4g

Carbohydrates: 19g

Protein: 14g

Spicy Chili Salmon

Serving: 4

Prep Time: 10 minutes

Cook Time: 7 minutes

Ingredients:

salmon fillets, boneless and skin-on

2 tablespoons assorted chili peppers, chopped Juice of 1 lemon

1 lemon, sliced

1 cup water

Black pepper

How To:

1.   Add water to the moment Pot.

2.   Add steamer basket and add salmon fillets, season the fillets with salt and pepper.

3.   Drizzle juice on top.

4.   Top with lemon slices.

5.   Lock the lid and cook on high for 7 minutes.

6.   Release the pressure naturally over 10 minutes.

7.   Divide the salmon and lemon slices between serving plates.

8.   Enjoy!

Nutrition (Per Serving)

Calories: 281

Fats: 8g

Carbs: 19g

Protein:7g

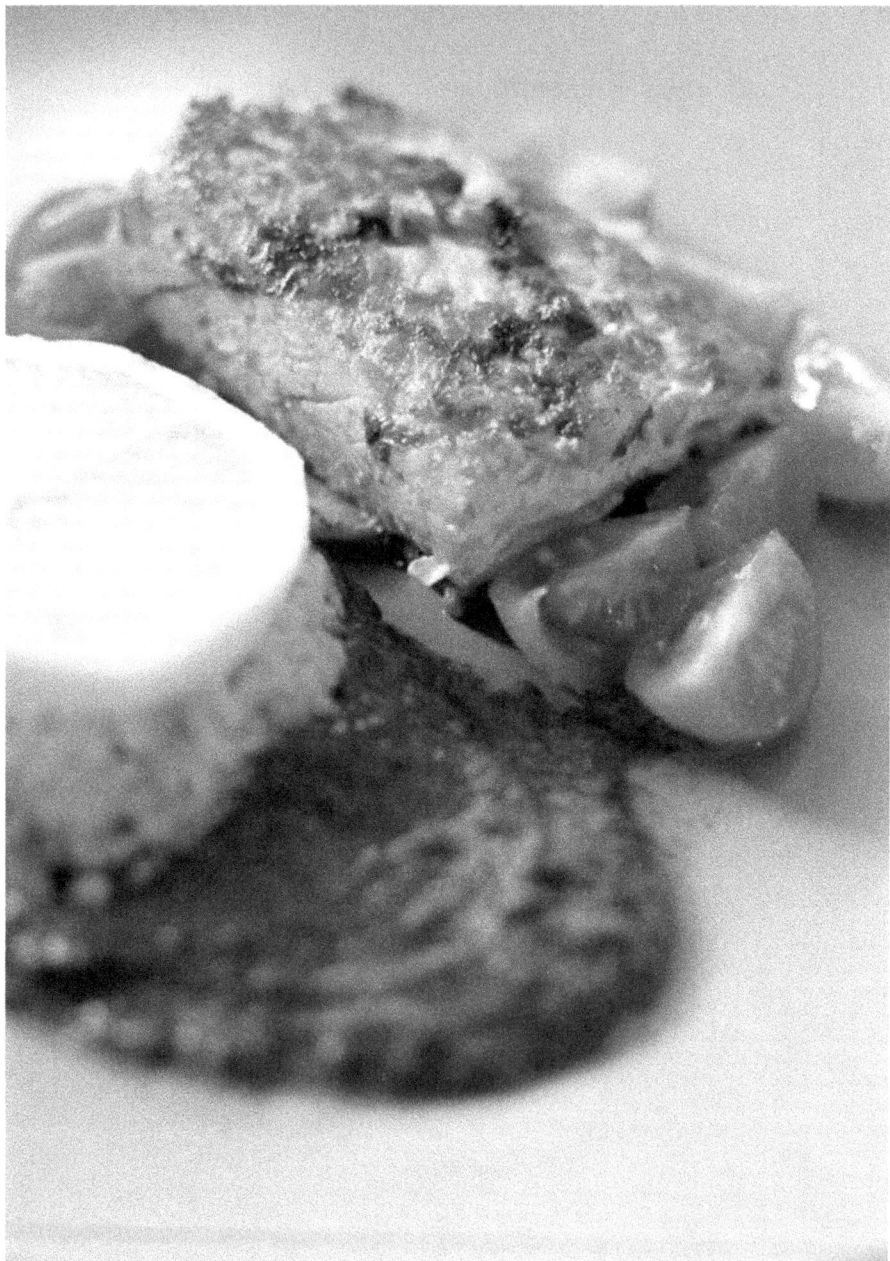

Niçoise Salad with Tuna Steak

Nutrition

Calories: 956 kcal | Gross carbohydrates: 6 g | Protein: 37 g |
Fats: 86 g |Fiber: 2 g | Net carbohydrates: 4 g | Macro fats: 68 %
| Macro proteins: 29 % |Macro carbohydrates: 3 %

Total time: 18 minutes

Ingredients

Tuna steaks

375 grams of tuna steaks If you use frozen food, defrost
beforehand.

3 tablespoons butter

Eggs

3 eggs

Vegetable

0.5 celeriac

90 grams of cherry tomatoes

180-gram haricot verts Drained weight - from a pot without
added sugar

1 bunch of radishes

1 tablespoon capers

3 tablespoons olives If you buy olives in oil, make sure they are
in olive oil and not in any other type of oil!

Dressing

300 ml mayonnaise

Instructions

1.   Eggs

2.   Start by boiling the eggs. Cook them in 8 minutes and then put them in a pan with cold water to cool.

3.   Peel and halve the eggs.

4.   Place the eggs on a large flat dish.

5.   Tuna steaks

6.   Melt the butter or ghee in a skillet or use a grill pan without butter.

7.   Cook the tuna in 2.5 minutes per side (or until cooked, depending on the thickness of the tuna steak).

8.   Place the tuna steaks on top of the haricot verts.

9.   Vegetable

10.   Use half a celery tuber. Cut the half tuber into 1.5 cm thick slices. Remove the skin and cut the slices into small cubes (approximately 1 cm -1.5 cm). Cook the cubes in the microwave or in a saucepan with some water. Allow to cool.

11.   Drain the haricot verts and then place them in the middle of the serving dish. Still have room for the celery tuber.

12.   Wash the tomatoes and halve them. Arrange them on the edge of the serving dish.

13.   Wash the radishes and halve them. Place them on the edge of the serving dish.

14.   Also, place the drained capers and olives on the edge of the serving dish.

15.   Arrange the celery tuber cubes next to the haricot verts.

16.   Sprinkle salt and pepper to taste over the eggs, tuna, and vegetables.

17.   Serve with mayonnaise or mix in the mayonnaise.

Whole Grain Pasta with Meat Sauce

Prep time: 10 minutes

Cook time: 30 minutes

Servings: 6

Ingredients

Whole-grain pasta – 1 pound

Extra-lean ground beef – 1 pound

Onion – 1, diced

Garlic – 3 cloves, minced

No-salt-added tomato sauce – 2 (8-ounce) cans

Red wine – 1/3 cup

Balsamic vinegar – 1 Tbsp.

Dried basil - 1 tsp.

Dried marjoram – ½ tsp.

Dried oregano – ½ tsp.

Dried red pepper flakes - ½ tsp.

Dried thyme - ½ tsp.

Freshly ground black pepper - ½ tsp.

Method

1.   Follow the direction on the package and cook the pasta. Omit the salt. Drain and set aside.

2.   Place onion, ground beef and garlic in a pan over medium heat. Stir-fry for 5 minutes, or until the beef has browned.

3.   Add remaining ingredients and stir to combine. Simmer, uncovered, for 10 minutes, stirring occasionally.

4.   Remove from heat and spoon over pasta.

5.   Serve.

Nutritional Facts Per Serving

Calories: 387

Fat: 5g

Carb: 58g

Protein: 27g

Sodium 65mg

Beef Tacos

Prep time: 10 minutes

Cook time: 20 minutes

Servings: 6

Ingredients

Extra-lean ground beef – 1 pound

Large onion – 1, chopped Garlic – 2 cloves, minced

No-salt-added tomato sauce – 1 (8-ounce) can Low-sodium

Worcestershire sauce – 2 tsp.

Molasses - 1 Tbsp.

Apple cider vinegar – 1 Tbsp.

Ground cumin – 1 Tbsp.

Ground sweet paprika – 1 Tbsp.

Dried red pepper flakes - ½ tsp.

Ground black pepper to taste

Low-sodium taco shells – 1 package

Chopped fresh cilantro - ¼ cup Tomato and lettuce of serving

Method

1.   Place the ground beef, onion, and garlic in a pan over medium heat.

2.   Stir-fry for 5 minutes or until the beef is browned.

3.   Lower heat to medium-low and add the Worcestershire sauce, tomato sauce, molasses, vinegar, cumin, red pepper flakes, paprika, and black pepper. Simmer, stirring frequently, about 10 minutes.

4.   Heat taco shells according to package directions. Set aside.

5.   Remove the sauté pan from the heat. Stir in cilantro.

6.   Divide evenly between the taco shells.

7.   Garnish with lettuce, tomato and serve.

Nutritional Facts Per Serving (2 tacos)

Calories: 255

Fat: 9g

Carb: 23g

Protein: 18g

Sodium 79mg

Dirty Rice

Prep time: 10 minutes

Cook time: 30 minutes

Servings: 4

Ingredients

Extra-lean ground beef - ½ pound

Large onion – 1, diced

Celery – 2 stalks, diced

Garlic – 2 cloves, minced

Bell pepper – 1, diced

Sodium-free beef bouillon granules - 1 tsp.

Water - 1 cup

Low-sodium Worcestershire sauce – 2 tsp.

Dried thyme – 1 ½ tsp.

Dried basil – 1 tsp.

Dried marjoram - ½ tsp.

Ground black pepper - ¼ tsp.

Pinch ground cayenne pepper

Scallions – 2, diced

Cooked long-grain brown rice – 3 cups

Method

1.	In a pan, place the onion, ground beef, celery, and garlic. Stir-fry for 5 minutes or until beef is browned.

2.	Add beef bouillon, bell pepper, water, sauce, and herbs and stir to combine.

3.	Bring to a boil.

4.	Then reduce heat to low, and cover.

5.	Simmer for 20 minutes.

6.	Stir in the scallions and simmer, uncovered, for 3 minutes.

7.	Remove from heat. Add cooked rice and stir to combine.

8.	Serve.

Nutritional Facts Per Serving

Calories: 272

Fat: 4g

Carb: 41g

Protein: 16g

Sodium 92mg

Healthy Berry Cobbler

Serving: 8

Prep Time: 10 minutes

Cooking Time: 2 hours 30 minutes

Ingredients:

1 ¼ cups almond flour

1 cup coconut sugar

1 teaspoon baking powder

½ teaspoon cinnamon powder

1 whole egg

¼ cup low-fat milk

2 tablespoons olive oil

2 cups raspberries

2 cups blueberries

How To:

1.   Take a bowl and add almond flour, coconut sugar, baking powder and cinnamon.

2.   Stir well.

3.   Take another bowl and add egg, milk, oil, raspberries, blueberries and stir.

4.   Combine both of the mixtures.

5.   Grease your Slow Cooker.

6.   Pour the combined mixture into your Slow Cooker and cook on HIGH for 2 hours 30 minutes.

7.   Divide between serving bowls and enjoy!

Nutrition (Per Serving)

Calories: 250

Fat: 4g

Carbohydrates: 30g

Protein: 3g

Tasty Poached Apples

Serving: 8

Prep Time: 10 minutes

Cooking Time: 2 hours 30 minutes

Ingredients:

6 apples, cored, peeled and sliced

1 cup apple juice, natural

1 cup coconut sugar

1 tablespoon cinnamon powder

How To:

1.   Grease Slow Cooker with cooking spray.

2.   Add apples, sugar, juice, cinnamon to your Slow Cooker.

3.   Stir gently.

4.   Place lid and cook on HIGH for 4 hours.

5.   Serve cold and enjoy!

Nutrition (Per Serving)

Calories: 180

Fat: 5g

Carbohydrates: 8g

Protein: 4g

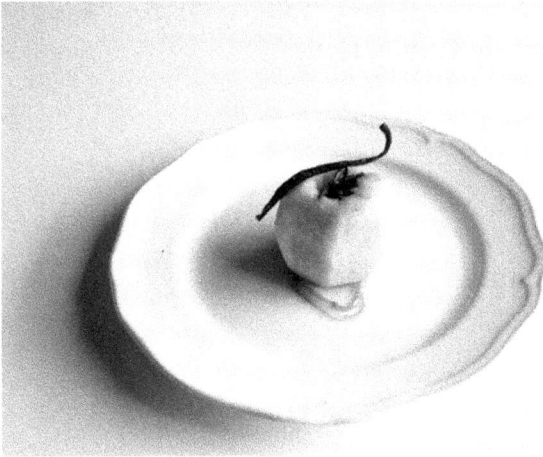

Home Made Trail Mix for The Trip

Serving: 4

Prep Time: 10 minutes

Cook Time: 55 minutes

Ingredients:

¼ cup raw cashews

¼ cup almonds

¼ cup walnuts

1 teaspoon cinnamon

2 tablespoons melted coconut oil

Sunflower seeds as needed

How To:

1.   Line baking sheet with parchment paper.

2.   Pre-heat your oven to 275 degrees F.

3.   Melt coconut oil and keep it on the side.

4.   Combine nuts to large mixing bowl and add cinnamon and melted coconut oil.

5.   Stir.

6.   Sprinkle sunflower seeds.

7.   Place in oven and brown for 6 minutes.

8.   Enjoy!

Nutrition (Per Serving)

Calories: 363

Fat: 22g

Carbohydrates: 41g

Protein: 7g

Heart Warming Cinnamon Rice Pudding

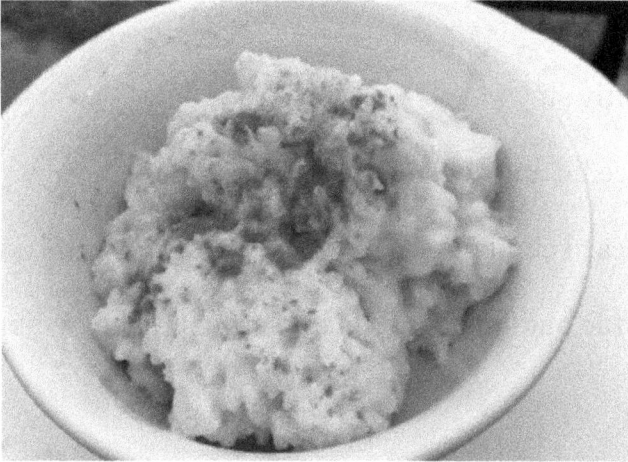

Serving: 4

Prep Time: 10 minutes

Cooking Time: 5 hours

Ingredients:

6 ½ cups water

1 cup coconut sugar

2 cups white rice

2 cinnamon sticks

½ cup coconut, shredded

How To:

1.   Add water, rice, sugar, cinnamon and coconut to your Slow Cooker.

2.   Gently stir.

3.   Place lid and cook on HIGH for 5 hours.

4.   Discard cinnamon.

5.   Divide pudding between dessert dishes and enjoy!

Nutrition (Per Serving)

Calories: 173

Fat: 4g

Carbohydrates: 9g

Protein: 4g

Pure Avocado Pudding

Serving: 4

Prep Time: 3 hours

Cook Time: nil

Ingredients:

1 cup almond milk

2 avocados, peeled and pitted

¾ cup cocoa powder

1 teaspoon vanilla extract

2 tablespoons stevia

¼ teaspoon cinnamon

Walnuts, chopped for serving

How To:

1.   Add avocados to a blender and pulse well.

2.   Add cocoa powder, almond milk, stevia, vanilla bean extract and pulse the mixture well.

3.   Pour into serving bowls and top with walnuts.

4.   Chill for 2-3 hours and serve!

Nutrition (Per Serving)

Calories: 221

Fat: 8g

Carbohydrates: 7g

Protein: 3g

Sweet Almond and Coconut Fat Bombs

Serving: 6

Prep Time: 10 minutes

Cooking Time: 10 minutes

Freeze Time: 20 minutes

Ingredients:

¼ cup melted coconut oil

9 ½ tablespoons almond butter

90 drops liquid stevia

3 tablespoons cocoa

9 tablespoons melted almond butter, sunflower seeds

How To:

1.   Take a bowl and add all of the listed ingredients.

2.   Mix them well.

3.   Pour 2 tablespoons of the mixture into as many muffin molds as you like.

4. Chill for 20 minutes and pop them out.

5. Serve and enjoy!

Nutrition (Per Serving)

Total Carbs: 2g

Fiber: 0g

Protein: 2.53g

Fat: 14g

Spicy Popper Mug Cake

Serving: 2

Prep Time: 5 minutes

Cook Time: 5 minutes

Ingredients:

2 tablespoons almond flour

1 tablespoon flaxseed meal

1 tablespoon almond butter

1 tablespoon cream cheese

1 large egg

1 bacon, cooked and sliced

½ jalapeno pepper

½ teaspoon baking powder

¼ teaspoon sunflower seeds

How To:

1.   Take a frying pan and place it over medium heat.

2.   Add slice of bacon and cook until it has a crispy texture.

3.   Take a microwave proof container and mix all of the listed ingredients (including cooked bacon), clean the sides.

4.   Microwave for 75 seconds, making to put your microwave to high power.

5.   Take out the cup and tap it against a surface to take the cake out.

6.   Garnish with a bit of jalapeno and serve!

Nutrition (Per Serving)

Calories: 429

Fat: 38g

Carbohydrates: 6g

Protein: 16g

Sensational Strawberry Medley

Serving: 2

Prep Time: 5 minutes

Ingredients:

1-2 handful baby greens

3 medium kale leaves

5-8 mint leaves

1-inch piece ginger , peeled

1 avocado

1 cup strawberries

6-8 ounces coconut water + 6-8 ounces filtered water Fresh juice of one lime

1-2 teaspoon olive oil

How To:

1. Add all the listed ingredients to your blender.

2. Blend until smooth.

3.   Add a few ice cubes and serve the smoothie.

4.   Enjoy!

Nutrition (Per Serving)

Calories: 200

Fat: 10g

Carbohydrates: 14g

Protein 2g

Mango's Gone Haywire

Serving: 2

Prep Time: 5 minutes

Ingredients:

1 mango, diced

2 bananas, diced

1-2 oranges, quartered

Dash of lemon juice

1 tablespoon hemp seed

¼ teaspoon green powder

Coconut water (as needed)

How To:

1. Add orange quarters in the blender first, blend.

2. Add the remaining ingredients and blend until smooth.

3. Add more coconut water to adjust the thickness.

4. Serve chilled!

Nutrition (Per Serving)

Calories: 200

Fat: 10g

Carbohydrates: 14g

Protein 2g

Unexpectedly Awesome Orange Smoothie

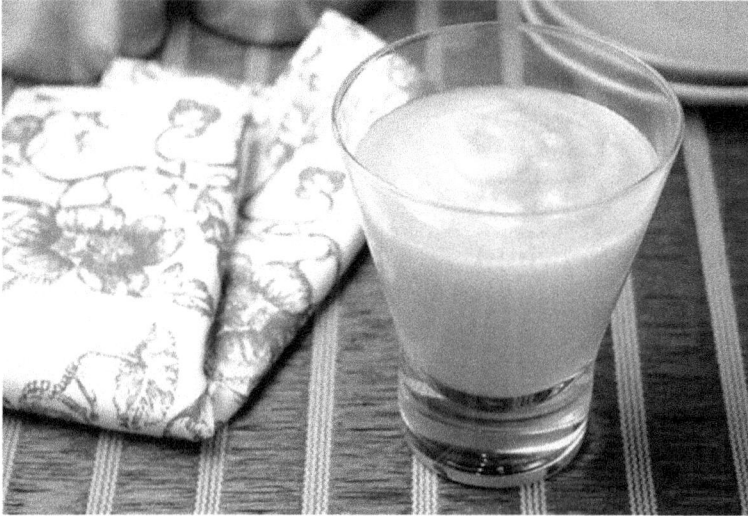

Serving: 2

Prep Time: 5 minutes

Ingredients:

1 orange, peeled

¼ cup fat-free yogurt

2 tablespoons frozen orange juice concentrate ¼ teaspoon vanilla extract

4 ice cubes

How To:

1.   Add the listed ingredients to your blender and blend until smooth.

2.   Serve chilled!

Nutrition (Per Serving)

Calories: 200

Fat: 10g

Carbohydrates: 14g

Protein 2g

Minty Cherry Smoothie

Serving: 2

Prep Time: 5 minutes

Ingredients:

¾ cup cherries

1 teaspoon mint

½ cup almond milk

½ cup kale

½ teaspoon fresh vanilla

How To:

1.   Wash and cut cherries.

2.   Take the pits out.

3.   Add cherries to blender.

4.   Pour almond milk.

5.   Wash the mint and put two sprigs in the blender.

6.   Separate the kale leaves from the stems.

7.   Put kale in blender.

8.   Press vanilla bean and cut lengthwise with knife.

9.   Scoop out your desired amount of vanilla and add to the blender.

10.   Blend until smooth.

11.   Serve chilled and enjoy!

Nutrition (Per Serving)

Calories: 200

Fat: 10g

Carbohydrates: 14g

Protein 2g

A Very Berry (and Green) Smoothie

Serving: 2

Prep Time: 5 minutes

Ingredients:

1 cup spinach leaves

½ cup frozen blueberries

1 ripe banana

½ cup milk

2 tablespoons old fashioned oats

½ tablespoon stevia

How To:

1.   Add the listed ingredients to your blender and blend until smooth.

2.   Serve chilled!

Nutrition (Per Serving)

Calories: 200

Fat: 10g

Carbohydrates: 14g

Protein 2g

Spicy Kale Chips

Serving: 4

Prep Time: 10 minutes

Cook Time: 25 minutes

Ingredients:

3 cups kale, stemmed and thoroughly washed, torn in 2-inch pieces

1 tablespoon extra-virgin olive oil

½ teaspoon chili powder

¼ teaspoon sea sunflower seeds

How To:

1.   Pre-heat your oven to 300 degrees F.

2.   Line 2 baking sheets with parchment paper and keep it on the side.

3.   Dry kale entirely and transfer to a large bowl.

4.   Add olive oil and toss.

5.   Make sure each leaf is covered.

6.   Season kale with chili powder and sunflower seeds, toss again.

7.   Divide kale between baking sheets and spread into a single layer.

8.   Bake for 25 minutes until crispy.

9.   Cool the chips for 5 minutes and serve.

10. Enjoy!

Nutrition (Per Serving)

Calories: 56

Fat: 4g

Carbohydrates: 5g

Protein: 2g

Seemingly Easy Portobello Mushrooms

Serving: 4

Prep Time: 10 minutes

Cook Time: 10 minutes

Ingredients:

12 cherry tomatoes

2 ounces scallions

4 portabella mushrooms

4 ¼ ounces almond butter

Sunflower seeds and pepper to taste

How To:

1.   Take a large skillet and melt almond butter over medium heat.

2.   Add mushrooms and sauté for 3 minutes.

3.   Stir in cherry tomatoes and scallions.

4.   Sauté for 5 minutes. 5. Season accordingly.

5. Sauté until veggies are tender.

6. Enjoy!

Nutrition (Per Serving)

Calories: 154

Fat: 10g

Carbohydrates: 2g

Protein: 7g

The Garbanzo Bean Extravaganza

Serving: 5

Prep Time: 10 minutes

Cook Time: Nil

Ingredients:

1 can garbanzo beans, chickpeas

1 tablespoon olive oil

1 teaspoon sunflower seeds

1 teaspoon garlic powder

½ teaspoon paprika

How To:

1.   Pre-heat your oven to 375 degrees F.

2.   Line a baking sheet with a silicone baking mat.

3.   Drain and rinse garbanzo beans, pat garbanzo beans dry and put into a large bowl.

4.   Toss with olive oil, sunflower seeds, garlic powder, paprika and mix well.

5.   Spread over a baking sheet.

6.   Bake for 20 minutes.

7.   Turn chickpeas so they are roasted well.

8.   Place back in oven and bake for another 25 minutes at 375 degrees F.

9.   Let them cool and enjoy!

Nutrition (Per Serving)

Calories: 395

Fat: 7g

Carbohydrates: 52g

Protein: 35g

Classic Guacamole

Serving: 6

Prep Time: 15 minutes

Cook Time: Nil

Ingredients:

3 large ripe avocados

1 large red onion, peeled and diced

4 tablespoons freshly squeezed lime juice Sunflower seeds as needed

Freshly ground black pepper as needed Cayenne pepper as needed

How To:

1.   Halve the avocados and discard stone.

2.   Scoop flesh from 3 avocado halves and transfer to a large bowl.

3.   Mash using a fork.

4.   Add 2 tablespoons of lime juice and mix.

5.   Dice the remaining avocado flesh (remaining half) and transfer to another bowl.

6.   Add remaining juice and toss.

7.   Add diced flesh with the mashed flesh and mix.

8.   Add chopped onions and toss.

9.   Season with sunflower seeds, pepper and cayenne pepper.

10.   Serve and enjoy!

Nutrition (Per Serving)

Calories: 172

Fat: 15g

Carbohydrates: 11g

Protein: 2g

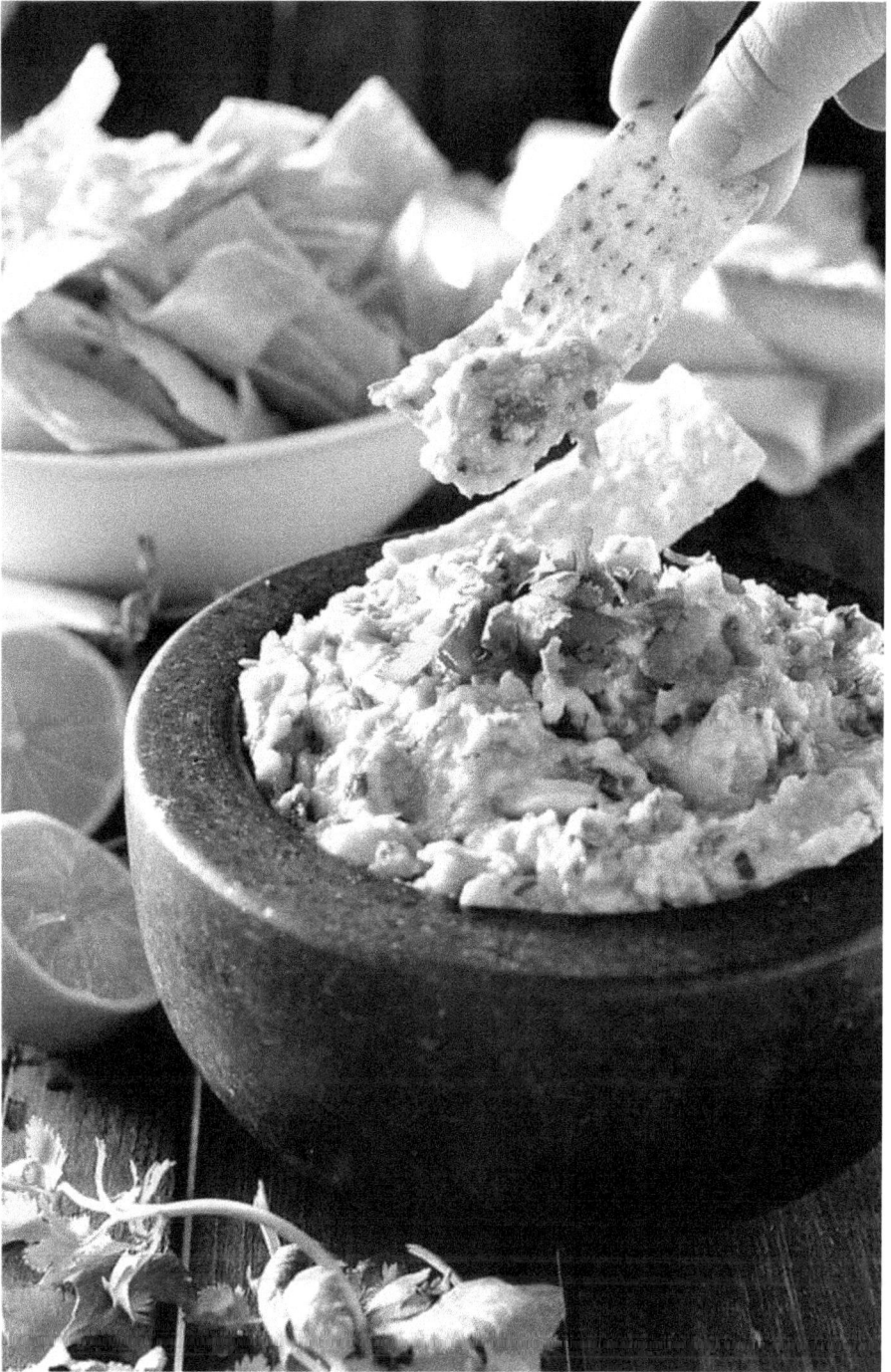

www.ingramcontent.com/pod-product-compliance
Lightning Source LLC
Chambersburg PA
CBHW050749030426
42336CB00012B/1733